THE FIELD MEDICS WORKBOOK

A PROVEN APPROACH FOR TRAINING PARAMEDICS

Samuel Adams and Christian Adams
NREMT Paramedics

Twin Peaks Publishing, LLC

www.Field-Medics.com

ISBN: Paperback: 978-0-9600337-2-0
EBook: 978-0-9600337-3-7

Contents

Introduction ____ 7

1

Benefit of This Workbook ____ 9

2

Training System ____ 13
- Knowledge ____ 14
- Interpersonal Skills and General Qualities ____ 14
- Decision-Making ____ 18
- The Role of the Preceptor Is Verification, not Re-Education ____ 21
- Learning Environment ____ 21
- Methodical Approach ____ 23
- Confidence and Independence ____ 26
- Building Confidence ____ 27

Methodical Approach ____ 31
- The Methodical Approach to a General Patient Assessment ____ 37
- Methodical Approach to Assessing the Respiratory Patient ____ 38
- SADRAP Simple Six ____ 38
- Every Respiratory Patient Gets Minimum ____ 39
- Methodical Approach for reading 12 lead EKG ____ 40

3

Decision-Making ____ 41

Decision-Making Worksheet ____ 45
- Factors that Affect Decision-Making ____ 47

4

Phase 1: Assimilation 51
- Step 1 55
- Expectations 59
- Step 2 61

Evaluation Forms 63
- Student/Candidate Self-Evaluation 63
- Medical Principles 64
- Interpersonal Skills 67
- Tools to Improve Skills 69
- Communication 69
- Teamwork 69
- Leadership 69
- Patient Assessment 70
- Delegation 70
- Setting the Tone (Tones 3 Cs) 70
- Qualities to Evaluate and Develop within Your Candidate 71
- Assessment of Qualities 73
- Step 3 78

Teaching Plans 79
- Complex Teaching Plan Objective 79
- Benchmarks to Meet the Goals 79
- Example—Teaching Plan 80
- Goals to Meet the Teaching Plan Objective: 80
- Benchmarks to Meet the Goals 81
- Step 4 86

5

Phase 2: Verification, Decision-Making, Leadership Development __ 87
Verification __ 87
Decision-Making __ 94
Leadership __ 97

6

Phase 3: Execution __ 105
Final Evaluation __ 106
Final Evaluation Form __ 111
About the Authors __ 113

Introduction

What is the purpose of this workbook? It's simple really. To give the paramedic who trains other paramedics a reliable, reproducible outline by which to train others.

It has taken a long time and many hours and many failures to develop a reproducible system to train others in the field. Training other paramedics is difficult. What makes it even more difficult is when you start from ground zero on every single trainee, whether they are a student or a candidate for field instruction.

Through the experience of training multiple students and putting multiple paramedics through a field instruction program, we have concluded that the only way to truly train someone is through a systematic approach. This realization came only after we floundered around with no real direction.

By using a systematic approach, it is easier to identify the qualities and skill sets needed in each student. Furthermore, a training program gives a clear understanding of what is being evaluated and how to evaluate each student.

Our approach can be tailored for the individual that you are training. Each individual will be different and will need different instruction. With a systematic approach, it will be easier for you, as preceptor, to identify what the trainee needs from you. It will be easier to identify the skill sets and qualities that you need to focus your attention on in order to bring out the best success in the person that you are training.

The primary purpose of this book, therefore, is to provide you, our colleagues in the field, with this proven approach to training paramedics.

How should you go about using this workbook? You need to use this workbook with the person that you are training. You should be well versed as the instructor in the different steps that are outlined here. You need to go over each step with your student and give them clear direction on what your expectations are.

We hope this workbook will be helpful. We invite your comments and experiences because in the classroom—and in the field—we all learn from each other.

1

Benefit of This Workbook

Why does a workbook like this benefit you as the instructor or preceptor (and we'll use those terms interchangeably to refer to you)? A guide is extremely beneficial because it gives you a systematic approach to train others. You cannot train others without any direction on where you are taking your student. You have to have a system in place on how to evaluate where someone's skills are currently, and how to get them to the finish line.

Such a systematic approach benefits you as the instructor because you will no longer be starting from square one with each new student. You now have a system that you can build upon and that you can tailor toward the unique needs of each individual student that you train. If you don't have a system in place, then you have nothing to tweak in order to meet the needs of your students.

This workbook gives you a starting point for training. Where do you begin? How do you evaluate someone? How do you assess the needs of your students? These questions and many others are easily answered if you start with a system that you can use repeatedly when training others. You will be able to communicate with your student what your expectations are. You will have a clear understanding of how to evaluate someone, and what skills you are actually looking for. By this we mean how you can tell if someone is capable of working independently as a paramedic.

Not a single instructor willingly puts trainees in the field that they do not believe are capable of meeting the expectations of a paramedic. It benefits you as an instructor to have a system in place so that the people that you train are more reliable, and you as the instructor are more reliable.

A training system should be simple enough that it is flexible. It needs this flexibility so that it can cater to the needs of all types of students. But a training system also needs to be comprehensive enough to give you, the instructor, a framework for how to proceed. This workbook provides a system that is an outline on how to train a paramedic.

The system presented here gives you the ability to evaluate growth. You will have a reliable, repeatable way to evaluate how your student is doing and the ability to identify what it is that your student is lacking. After identifying the needs of your students, you will be more capable of addressing them. With a training outline, you will become a much better instructor, and you will be infinitely more effective at training others.

Another benefit of having a systematic approach is not only for you, but it is for your student. Your student will absolutely grow faster in their understanding of what they're supposed to be doing as a new paramedic. A systematic approach will give them clearly defined expectations and evaluations. Your student will be able to grow much faster because there will not be any sort of misunderstanding between you as the instructor, and them, of what it is that you want from them.

The ultimate beneficiary of this systematic approach will be the patients we all serve. If you start early with students on the importance of being systematic and methodical, such an approach will lead to better patient care.

2

Training System

The first step in developing a system that can be used to train others is to clearly define the philosophy behind the system that we will implement.

The primary theme behind the system will be integration. In order to develop a paramedic, we must integrate these three areas:

1. Knowledge or educational understanding
2. Interpersonal skills and general qualities
3. Decision-making

As preceptors, we need to focus on developing all three of these skills in the individual candidates so they can become more successful and provide high-quality patient care.

Knowledge

Let's begin with the first principle of knowledge.

Knowledge is what is gained through paramedic school and through other courses taken that are required of a paramedic in order to provide patient care. This is where paramedics gain the clinical understanding of disease processes and how your interventions work on them. This knowledge comes from lots of study, reading, and classwork in order to gain the proper insight and clinical understanding to treat patients.

Knowledge is a key factor that paramedics must have in order to properly treat people. Knowledge is the instrument that drives decision-making, which is why it must be integrated with decision-making. **Decision-making must be integrated with interpersonal skills such as communication and teamwork in order to implement the paramedic's vision for patient care.** All of this, however, starts with a foundation of clinical knowledge, which can then be applied to what is going on with the patient. Gaining knowledge is a never-ending process that lasts the entire career for every paramedic.

Interpersonal Skills and General Qualities

The second principle we integrate is interpersonal skills. Interpersonal skills must be integrated into decision-making, which is driven from knowledge. We briefly define a few interpersonal skills that you should look for in your students.

> **Communication**. Communication is vitally important for the paramedic. You must develop this understanding with your student. Your student must display the ability to communicate properly with your patient, with your team, and with bystanders or witnesses. If you identify a problem in communication, you must work to build

their communication skills so they can implement their vision for treatment plans.

Teamwork. Teamwork is another critical interpersonal skill that must be evaluated. Is your student able to work within a team effectively? Does your student understand that they are working in a team and that they are not the only one who is implementing their treatment plan? Does your student display the ability to utilize team members effectively? Does your student routinely consider the ideas of other team members for treatment plans? These questions should be considered and evaluated when you have a new student.

Leadership. Another critical interpersonal skill that must be evaluated is leadership. Does your student display the ability to lead other people? Does your student display the ability to delegate tasks to other team members? Does your student have the ability to identify what their vision is for a treatment plan and then effectively communicate that to other team members? Your student's leadership capabilities should be evaluated.

Assessment skills. Assessment skills are a demonstration of a paramedic's ability to gain vital information and then determine what medical problems the patient may be suffering from. Your student's assessment skills are also a direct representation of their interpersonal skills.

Assessment skills must be developed and maintained with your students. How does the candidate talk to your patient, talk with the team, and talk with bystanders? Assessment skills are by definition a reflection of their ability to communicate with others. You must evaluate your student's assessment skills in light of their knowledge, and their interpersonal skills such as communication. They must be integrated in order to provide the best quality patient care.

These are some primary interpersonal skills that must be evaluated in order to properly identify the needs of your students. If your student lacks any of these interpersonal skills, then you must address them and create a teaching plan for them to improve these interpersonal skills.

Next, we look for and integrate into our system a student's general qualities. There are many different qualities that the paramedic should exhibit. Here we list a few of those qualities.

> **Integrity**. Does your student display integrity? A brief definition of integrity might help. Does your student do what is right even when no one is looking? Do you question whether or not your student has integrity? Do you question whether they are doing what is right for the patient? Do you question whether they will continue to provide good patient care even when you're not around? Do you question whether your student cares about the general well-being of their patients? A couple examples of a breach in integrity would be lying about patient care, making excuses for decisions made, or blaming others for treatment plans.

A brief evaluation of your student's integrity and then integrating that into the training system will greatly benefit you and the student.

> **Compassion**. Does your student demonstrate compassion? Are they compassionate with their patients? Are there certain types of patients that they are less compassionate with? This doesn't mean that they're doing anything wrong; this just means that you

are intentionally trying to identify whether they are consistently displaying compassion.

If you identify a specific type of patient that your student is not compassionate with, it might be something that you want to identify with them and then have a talk with them about. If your student is cold and callous toward every single person that they interact with, that is something you should address. On the whole, your students should be compassionate toward all the people they are treating.

Accountability. Does your student demonstrate and take accountability for their actions? Are they accountable to themselves? And are they accountable to you? If you find that your student is not accountable to themselves or to you as the preceptor, you should address it.

Accountability must be integrated into the training system. Your student must understand that they will be held accountable for the treatment plans and any interventions that they perform. This must be understood by your student and addressed by you as their instructor.

Responsibility. Is your student responsible? Do they understand what they are responsible for now that they are a paramedic? They are now responsible for implementing more complex treatment plans. They are responsible for providing high-quality patient care to the citizens they serve. They are responsible for knowing the protocols and guidelines that they are using. They're responsible for maintaining their equipment, to include, specifically, any controlled substances and paralytics. There are many new responsibilities for a new paramedic, and these should be formally addressed by you, the instructor.

Intent. Intent is a quality that should be developed and defined with your student. We will define intention as decisiveness with purpose. Does your student execute treatment plans with intention? Do they make decisions with clear purpose behind them? Do they demonstrate intention behind their actions?

Decision-Making

The last principle to focus on is decision-making. You must understand that you are not training somebody to regurgitate information. The primary focus of your training and instruction of your student should be developing a decision-making process. It is not to teach the medicine. It is teaching decision-making. Does your student demonstrate a sound decision-making process? Are they capable of making good decisions in chaotic environments?

For purposes of prehospital medicine, a good decision is acting in accordance with the standard of care that your medical directors have set forth and by providing high-quality treatment plans to your patient in a timely manner. A good decision made by your candidate is a decision that is made independent from your input as the instructor. It is a decision that reflects proper understanding of treatment guidelines and medical principles and also taking into consideration the patient's best interests.

What drives your student's decision-making? Here is a brief list of factors that influence decision-making. Understand that the primary factor that drives all decision-making is information. Which is why information must be integrated into your student's decision-making process.

Information. Does your student correctly interpret the information that they're gaining from their assessment and then implement the correct treatment plan?

Experience. Is your student already experienced and are they able to use that experience to supplement their decision-making? Experience does not drive decision-making; it supplements decision-making. Experience is absolutely necessary. However, running calls mindlessly with no clear objective or intention behind it is not nearly as productive. Your student needs a defined objective on calls in order to gain the proper experience. The most important of which is the experience of making decisions. It's not just gaining experience for the sake of experience.

Objectivity. Are they objective? Is your student able to remain objective to the information that they're gaining and then use that objectivity to create good decisions?

Flexibility. Is your student flexible? Are they able to change treatment plans on the fly? Are they able to gather new information and change treatment plans based on new information they are getting? Are they able to correctly evaluate team members' input and implement that into their treatment plan? Flexibility is something that should be stressed when it comes to decision-making. You need to help foster and develop this within your student.

These are a few factors that influence decision-making. Take the time to understand what these factors are. Are there any other factors that you believe are important to inform decisions? Those factors are important and you should define them clearly. Creating a sound, reliable, and consistent decision-making process is the single most important factor that a paramedic must have. You must stress this with your student.

You must stress that their decision-making is a direct reflection of their understanding of medical principles. Additionally, their decision-making, or lack thereof, is a direct representation of the student's willingness to take responsibility and accountability for their actions.

When your student is demonstrating to you that they are willing to take responsibility for their actions and responsibility for their treatment plans, it is telling you that they understand the consequences of their actions.

We have defined the three areas of focus that you should evaluate. These three areas are what you as the trainer should look to integrate into your student. Here is an example of how these three are integrated into one tool:

Your **communication** skills are used to assess your patient. The information you gain from the assessment is then filtered through your **knowledge** of medical principles. That filtered information then drives you to make a **decision** on what the treatment plan is. That **vision** you have for your treatment plan is then realized by leading your team in **implementing** it. Then you **delegate** to team members tasks needed in order to accomplish your vision for the **treatment of the patient**.

Work on integrating and developing all of these concepts for building more successful paramedics. Do not focus only on the student's medical knowledge. These three principles of knowledge, interpersonal skills, and decision-making, need to be integrated in order to begin the framework of the systematic approach.

The Role of the Preceptor Is Verification, not Re-Education

Verify your student's knowledge. Do not reteach them everything that they have already proven proficiency in paramedic school. Keep in mind that if they're interning with you, they've already demonstrated a certain level of competency. They've already demonstrated their ability to interpret 12 leads, demonstrated their ability to understand pharmacology, and demonstrated their ability to perform certain skills.

Now your role as preceptor is to guide the student in the *application* of those skills and knowledge. You want to mold their thought process. You want to take those medical principles and show them how to apply them in the field—to develop the student's decision-making process and methodical approach.

As specific situations arise, certainly pause and ensure that the student specifically understands that situation (Example: Student has been instructed on how a COPD exacerbation patient may present, but may have never seen one. Pause for a second and ensure they understand.). This allows the candidate to put into context the information that they have learned and that they must apply. This type of learning reinforces the candidate's understanding.

Learning Environment

What is the learning environment? Make sure that you create a learning environment that affords the student every opportunity for success. Your student should be comfortable and calm and feel confident in their ability to communicate with you as their preceptor.

Create an environment where the student is determined and confident in their own abilities, their abilities to make decisions, and their abilities to discuss situations with you. You have to create a proper learning environment so that they can learn and be successful.

So how do you create the proper learning environment? Communication is the key. Your student has to be comfortable communicating with you. Keep in mind that you as the preceptor probably function within another team, so allow the student the opportunity to assimilate with the team. They also have to feel comfortable communicating with the other people in your team.

Expectations is also a pivotal *must* in order to properly create a good learning environment. You must develop expectations for yourself and for your student or candidate. You will then articulate and inform your student of the expectations. This creates a degree of trust and understanding between the preceptor and trainee. Now there are no hidden agendas or unknowns. Everything is out in the open with no surprises. This lessens the anxiety and helps to establish a comfortable learning environment.

This next part is a key factor for the learning environment. The way you actually create it is by getting out of your student's way. You must allow your student to demonstrate to you that they can apply the knowledge that they have acquired. So how do you do this?

It is really actually very simple. Shut your mouth as the instructor, put your ego in the closet, or better yet just lose it, and let your students treat patients. Now, obviously, if you need to intervene for safety purposes and patient care, then do so, but those should be about the only reasons you intervene and change a treatment plan.

If your student wants to give pain medications to a patient, then allow them to do it, even if you wouldn't. That's the key. They must be able and comfortable to make their own decisions and execute their own treatment plans. You should very rarely tell your student, "I would do this," or "I wouldn't do that, but if you want to." Your goal is to create a learning environment where your student never really knows what you would or would not do on a scene.

If you as the instructor can do that, then you have succeeded to some degree in creating that ideal learning environment. This does take time, however, and a steadfast resolve on the part of the instructor. It will take around 100 to 150 hours for your student to start to trust that you won't "kneecap" them and change a treatment plan or start intervening and directing the call.

So what does this mean? It means you as the instructor must sit back and give your student the latitude to work. If you can do this, the student's learning curve will improve drastically, because now they are learning about how they interpret information, categorize it, prioritize it, and then execute their own treatment plans. They are not learning how you do it, and then mimic you; they are doing it themselves, which gives them an extremely beneficial environment and makes them much more capable.

At the end of the day, what this environment means for you, as the instructor, is a lot more work. More medications given potentially, more ride-ins to the hospital, if applicable, more refusals done. Longer hours talking with your student about why they chose to do whatever they chose to do, and never giving them a so-called Scooby-Snack and telling them what to do and how you would do it. They must be able to articulate to you the treatment plans that they chose and why.

Methodical Approach

Let's quickly review what the methodical approach is (and also refer to the workbook section A following this discussion). The methodical approach is the method that you use to assess a specific patient. For example, you may assess a respiratory patient the same way every single time looking for specific signs and symptoms and asking specific questions. That's your method. Now keep in mind that your method should be implemented consistently with every single respiratory patient. It becomes your methodical approach toward assessing a specific patient.

We now explore one of the most pivotal points in creating and developing a new paramedic. The methodical approach is the starting point for developing a paramedic's decision-making process. This is the point where the student begins to have buy-in on what it is that they're actually trying to accomplish. The methodical approach that you as the preceptor develop with your student is their own approach to specific patients. Now keep in mind that the methodical approach has to be employed and implemented consistently on every single patient or on every single specific call.

Developing these approaches early in the process of precepting does a couple of things. It allows you to have a basic understanding of where the student is. Where their own comfort level is. And what sort of processes they have already thought through. This also gives them a tangible template by which to act. Then you can implement that approach consistently on those patients, and it reveals inadequacies within that approach.

Then, after implementing that approach, mold it to be more substantive and effective. If you do this at the beginning of the preceptorship or the internship, you have more time to analyze whether or not it is effective and you will have more time to build and refine it. You're not mandating that the student implement your methodical approach; you're helping them develop *their* methodical approach.

When a new paramedic is beginning an internship, sit down with your student and discuss a few scenarios that you develop an approach for. An approach should be developed for each of these five basic patients:

1. Method for basic approach to a call
2. Method for assessing the cardiac patient
3. Method for the respiratory patient
4. Method for the trauma patient
5. Method for the general illness patient

Next, discuss reflection. Reflection, keep in mind, is a common theme throughout the internship. You're going to be reflecting on lots of different aspects of paramedicine throughout the internship. The methodical approach is no different. You must reflect on the methodical approaches that you develop with your students. You have to reflect on the efficiency and the effectiveness of those approaches.

As you're reflecting on the approach, then you can determine whether or not the student is accomplishing what you want them to accomplish. And then, after reflecting, you can tweak certain areas within the approach and fine-tune it.

For the methodical approach to truly be effective and developed during the internship, you have to keep in mind that the students should be given the liberty to develop their own approaches. You're there to mold, guide, and direct where the approach is going. Don't require the student to assess patients in a way that is unnatural for them. They should be comfortable with their approach. It should be a natural progression that they're implementing, not a forced one. That's why you as the preceptor have to give them the liberty, and you have to work with them to develop it.

Confidence and Independence

From discipline to execution and everything in between. This is really what we are trying to get at. We are trying to develop paramedics who are self-disciplined and can execute proper and high-quality treatment plans. The student will go through a number of stages to realize that they can and will execute good treatment plans.

The first stage is self-discipline. You must instill a sense of self-discipline within your student. This will drive them to be a better paramedic. Self-discipline then drives your student to operate and prepare with intention and determination. Now they are not arbitrarily or whimsically preparing with no purpose. They are preparing a methodical approach with the intention and determination of providing high-quality patient care every single time.

Because they are prepared, they can consistently start to implement good treatment plans. Through this consistency they realize that what they are doing is now reliable. The reliability gives them confidence that what they're doing is working and that they are providing quality patient care.

After they realize that what they are doing is reliable and they are consistently implementing it, now they must be disciplined to continue to implement it. This sequence creates habits and instills a high degree of personal confidence. These stages are how you develop good habits within your students.

Once they are implementing consistent treatment plans and discover that those treatment plans are reliable, they are developing these techniques to be a habit within themselves. Now your student is able to execute the treatment plan as needed in order to provide quality patient care. Let's go through this one more time.

The training process starts with self-discipline, which drives intention and determination. Intention and determination drive preparation. Preparation now drives confidence in the ability to start to apply knowledge. These steps now must be done consistently, which then drives reliability. Reliability then drives habits, and habits drive execution.

Now your student and you as the instructor should be able to go to calls and recognize very quickly what's taking place and how to execute a good quality treatment plan—because now you both have a reliable and consistent method by which to interpret information, categorize information, prioritize skills and interventions, and then execute a treatment plan.

Building Confidence

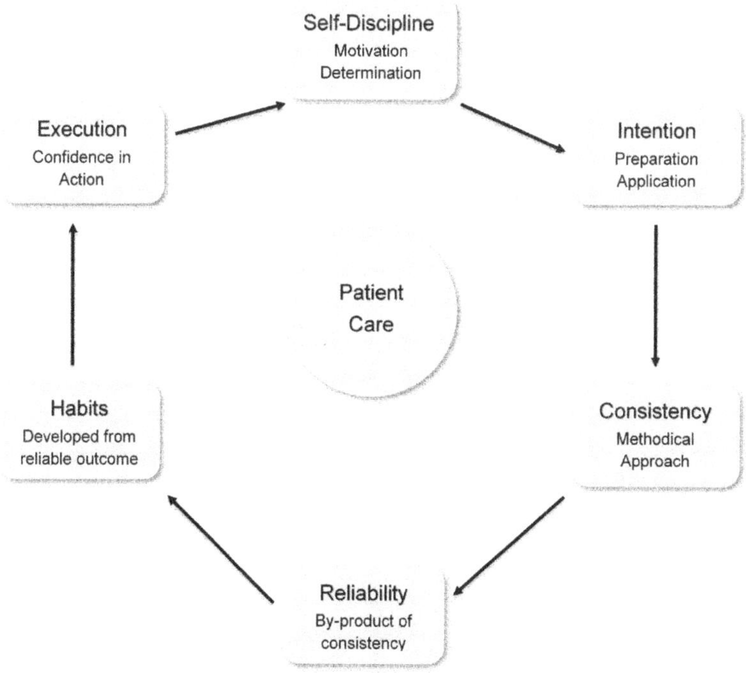

Workbook

The workbook sections appear in the text where you would implement them. We encourage you to go to the book's website at www.Field-Medics.com and download these as blank forms and checklists to use with your students.

Methodical Approach

During phases 1 and 2 (as explained in future chapters), you will be developing methods in three distinct areas with your student/candidate. Developing these methods early on in the instruction and applying them consistently creates a reliable process for patient care and, in turn, creates confidence for your candidate. These areas are as follows:

1. Methods for patient assessment. (How does the student as an individual provider assess these patients? Do they gather information consistently? What signs and symptoms are they looking for specifically?)
    a. Respiratory patient
    b. Cardiac patient

   c. Trauma patient
   d. General illness patient
   e. Basic approach to a call

2. Methods for interpreting information
   a. 12 lead EKG
   b. Capnography
   c. Vital signs
   d. Physical findings
      i. Breath sounds
      ii. Abdominal findings
      iii. Skin signs
      iv. Anatomical deformities
      v. Apparent life threats

3. Methods for performing interventions and skills
   a. CPAP
   b. Airway skills and management
      i. Intubation
      ii. Cricothyrotomy
      iii. BLS skills
      iv. Supraglottic airway device
      v. RSI (if applicable)
   c. IVs, IOs, and EJs
   d. Medication administration
      i. Drip sets
      ii. IV pushes

e. Cardiac monitor
    i. Defibrillation
    ii. Pacing
    iii. Sync cardioversion
    iv. Other basic functions
f. Bandaging
g. Bleeding control
h. Splinting
i. Capnography

During phases 1 and 2 each of the following subjects needs at minimum one day of concentrated focus and instruction.

1. Mental status exam
    a. How to methodically assess the mental status
2. Cardiology and chest pain
    a. 12 lead EKG interpretation; STEMI identification; Hyper K+
    b. Rhythm identification and treatment of said rhythm on a rhythm generator
        i. Develops and reinforces the flexibility of treatment
        ii. Reinforces decision-making abilities in low-stress environment
        iii. Builds leadership and communication skills in a low-stress environment
3. Respiratory patient
    a. Identification of the difficulty breathing patient
    b. CPAP

c. Capnography
d. Cricothyrotomy
e. Intubation
f. BLS airways
g. Lung sounds
h. Treatment plans
    i. COPD
    ii. CHF
    iii. Asthma
    iv. Anaphylaxis
    v. Trauma
    vi. Pneumonia

4. Refusals
    a. Criteria (based on provider guidelines or protocols)
    b. Mental status

5. Pediatrics
    a. Airway
    b. Croup
    c. Epiglottitis
    d. Needle cricothyrotomy
    e. Broselow tape or similar device
    f. Medication administration
    g. Choking
    h. Pediatric arrest

6. Trauma
    a. Methodical physical exam
    b. Traumatic arrest
    c. Needle decompression
    d. Wound packing and bandaging
    e. Tourniquets
    f. Airway management
    g. Multisystem trauma
    h. Splinting
    i. Spinal immobilization

As described, the methodical approach is essential to the success of your paramedic candidate. You must take the time to develop your candidate's methods of action in order to ensure they are successful and have a solid foundation when moving on and functioning in an independent capacity.

Methods can change from individual to individual; however, defining a few key aspects of a method may be beneficial when starting out. These are for both you, the instructor, and to develop within your student. Each individual provider should understand these concepts for themselves.

- You must understand what information you are trying to attain.
- You must understand how to attain that information (through assessment questions or physical exams).
- You must understand how you interpret that information.
- You must understand how you categorize and prioritize that information.
- You must understand how you execute a plan to address the priorities.

Notice that these concepts are brief and unspecific, but each principle can be applied to every call and every situation. Understanding these concepts and then defining methods for your specific patient will greatly benefit you and your candidate.

Here are a few examples of a methodical approach. These, keep in mind, are examples. Each individual provider is responsible for developing their own methodical approach toward patient care in accordance with individual protocols, guidelines, and scope of practice. Implementing methods consistently is crucial for success, reliability, and ultimately confidence for both the instructor and the candidate.

The Methodical Approach to a General Patient Assessment

Arrive on scene and make patient contact.

SICK

Sick patients from now on will be defined as being in need of IMMEDIATE lifesaving intervention (airway, breathing, major bleeding control, scene hazards).

NOT SICK

This is defined as a patient who does NOT require immediate lifesaving intervention. Slow down and assess your patient through your interview and exam. This is the majority of the patients you see.

Determine the chief complaint.

Take vital signs and gather information through assessment.

Interpret the information and develop differentials.

Categorize differentials into probable vs. possible.

Prioritize probable as working diagnosis.

Develop your treatment plan and vision for patient care and prioritize interventions.

Execute your plan and vision.

Reassess your plan and vision for success and efficacy.

This methodical approach can be applied to every call—ensuring that the vision remains the same for patient care regardless of the complaint.

Methodical Approach to Assessing the Respiratory Patient

Arrive on scene and make patient contact.

SICK

Requires IMMEDIATE lifesaving intervention (airway, ventilations, CPR).

NOT SICK

Keep in mind the not-sick may still be critically ill; however, a more detailed assessment takes place. This is the vast majority of your patients.

SADRAP Simple Six

Skin (pale, clammy, cool, HOT, rash, hives)

Audible sounds (across the room: stridor, wheezing, gurgling, coughing)

Dyspnea (can the patient speak comfortably between breaths)

Rate (respiratory rate, fast, slow, normal)

Accessory muscles (supraclavicular muscle use noted, intercostals)

Position (tripod, sniffing, supine, anxious, and uncomfortable)

The **SADRAP SIMPLE SIX** is used CONSISTENTLY. Learn how to interpret the information the patient is SHOWING you.

Every Respiratory Patient Gets Minimum

- Vital signs with room air sat or home O2 sat if possible
- ETCO2 — ETCO2 — ETCO2 (interpret methodically)
- LUNG SOUNDS (listen methodically)
- 12 lead (interpret information and categorize/prioritize 12 lead — interpret methodically)
- Gather history of present illness
- **Interpret information** and develop differentials.
- **Categorize information** and differentials to probable vs. possible.
- **Prioritize** treatments and working diagnosis.
- Develop a treatment plan and vision for patient care.
- **Execute** treatment plan and vision.
- **Reevaluate** your treatment plan and vision.

Methodical Approach for reading 12 lead EKG

AHI – AHI:

- r**A**te
- r**H**ythm
- **I**nterval
- **A**xis
- **H**ypertrophy, **H**yper K+
- **I**nfarct

3

Decision-Making

Decision-making is probably the key factor that exemplifies a successful paramedic. Decision-making involves all aspects of training and qualities within the paramedic. Decision-making should be your primary focus as the instructor (also refer to the Workbook—Decision-Making Worksheet at the end of this chapter).

Developing decision-making within your student is your primary goal. Decision-making involves many different aspects. And a lot of different factors drive decision-making.

The number one consideration that drives decision-making is information—information that must be gained through the patient assessment. That information is then filtered through your student's educational knowledge. Then after filtering the information gained through knowledge, the student is able to act decisively. This is an example of why teaching an integrated understanding of patient care is so valuable to you as an instructor, rather than focusing on the one primary area of didactic understanding of medical principles.

You can focus on and develop many other areas with the student. These other areas will improve the student's confidence, which in turn will make them more decisive. Avoid conversations of "Well this is what I would do" or " I do this." Instead, focus on why they did what they did. If you provide them all the answers of what you would do, they do not learn decision-making independent from your input; all they learn is how to please you, their instructor.

Here is a brief list of different factors that drive decision-making in your student:

- **Information.** Gather information in order to inform their decisions.
- **Education.** Filter information through their understanding of medicine.
- **Experience.** Used correctly and humbly will inform their decisions and give them confidence. Do not, however, let the student become overconfident.
- **Intuition.** Developed after reflecting on critical and noncritical incidents. Intuition informs and develops their experience so it is now valuable. Must be developed, does not just happen.
- **Objectivity.** Are they remaining objective about the information gathered by their assessment? Don't make the information say something it doesn't in order to fit a certain bias.
- **Flexibility.** Ability to change treatment plans confidently. Ability to utilize the team's input and incorporate that into the treatment plan.
- **Consistency and Reliability.** Making good decisions consistently and then understanding those decisions will produce reliability.

Decision-Making Worksheet

Rate your candidates according to the following scale:

1 Candidate demonstrates no ability to take decisive action. Candidate routinely asks for guidance and prompting. No decision is made independent of instructor input.

3 Candidate demonstrates the ability to make decisions but routinely hesitates and delays treatment because of uncertainty. Meets the bare minimum for providing the standard of care.

5 Candidate demonstrates the ability to act decisively with no input from the instructor. Candidate is making decisions independently and implementing vision with no instructor input.

Decisive

1 2 3 4 5

Assertive

1 2 3 4 5

Confident

1 2 3 4 5

Identify a critical call and break it down. These lists can be exhaustive. The more time and effort put into understanding the decisions made on calls will greatly improve the student in four major ways.

1. Builds and reinforces their understanding of medical principles already learned.
2. Gives them confidence they are correctly filtering the information through their medical understanding.
3. Builds and develops leadership skills such as delegation and communication.
4. Develops an understanding of the student's individual process for gathering and interpreting information and how they make decisions. This then makes them more consistent and then consistency produces reliability. Routine reflection forces the student to demonstrate the principles of interpreting

information, categorizing information, prioritizing interventions, and executing treatment plans.

Answering these questions allows you as the preceptor to more easily determine if your candidate is making bad decisions and why and subsequently create a plan to address it.

- What was the nature of the call?
- What was the outcome?
- What were the interventions performed?
- What factors contributed to the student's decisions made on the call? Identify what the student saw that drove them to make the decisions they made and then allow the student the ability to articulate their reasoning.
- Was it an emergent return to the hospital? Why or why not?
- Why did you perform the interventions you did? Focus on why the intervention was performed, not on the intervention itself. What did the student see to cause them to intervene?
- Did the decision improve the patient's outcome?
- Are these decisions and assessments able to be used to reinforce or create a methodical approach to the patient type that is being examined?

Factors that Affect Decision-Making

This next section is composed of multiple factors that affect decision-making on an emergency scene. If your candidate is having difficulty making decisions independent of instructor prompt or input, refer to this section. These factors here will be briefly discussed and can help to narrow down why your candidate might be having difficulty.

Information. Does the candidate gather too little or too much information prior to acting? Are they misinterpreting the information? Are they not capable of filtering the information through their understanding of medical principles? This is what we would call application.

Experience. How much experience does the candidate have? Are they relying too much on previous experience? Are they overconfident with perceived experience that they are making rash decisions too quickly without fully evaluating the situation? On every call you run with the candidate, build their experience by going through the call in depth. There is much to learn on even the basic calls.

Logic and Reason. Is your candidate acting reasonably for the situations that they find themselves in? Do they quickly become overwhelmed and throw their logical conclusions to the wind and start acting irrationally? Are they making decisions that are founded in emotional response to a situation or are they able to detach from a critical situation, evaluate, and then reengage with decisive action? This can be taught if it is formally addressed.

Gut Feeling or Intuition. Experience informs intuition. This is how intuition is developed. Is your candidate able to recognize patterns and common themes with the patients that they are providing care to? Develop the candidate's intuition through general and self-reflection of the experiences that they are now having. This helps your candidate anticipate patient needs in the future.

Intuition is extremely beneficial to decision-making if properly utilized.

Objectivity. Is your candidate remaining objective to the information that they are gathering? Are they making decisions based on a preconceived notion as to what might be taking place? Remaining objective is the key to flexible treatment plans and decisive action. Is your candidate allowing personal feelings or emotions to dictate decisions, or are they objective to the situation in front of them?

Subjectivity. Does your candidate allow time for the patient to inform them what is going on? Do they disregard subjective information that the patient says? Is your candidate too concerned with "finding the faker" that they don't act when they should? Is your candidate cocky and overconfident so they don't believe the patient and then fail to advocate?

Personal Factors. Does workload affect your candidate's decision-making? Are they concerned with writing patient reports? Are they concerned about having to ride into the hospital if certain interventions are done? If this comes up, it is a lack of self-discipline and must be addressed.

Consistency, Reliability, and the Methodical Approach. Is the candidate implementing the methods that you have helped them develop? Do they run each call as if it's the first time they are interacting with a patient? These concepts are all integrated.

Open to New Information. Does your candidate demonstrate the ability to incorporate new information into their treatment plan? Can they digest new information and act accordingly? Are they constantly looking for new information? They should be. This is the ongoing assessment. Or do they set it and forget it, so to speak?

Flexibility. New information is directly related to flexibility. Flexibility is broader, however. Is your candidate flexible? With treatment plans? With environments? With teammates? With constructive criticism? Or are they rigid with blinders on and no ability to recognize that a treatment plan needs to change?

Outside Influence. Does your candidate easily allow the outside influence of other teammates to change a proper treatment plan? Incorporating team members is important, but the student cannot let input negatively affect treatment plans. Do they allow patient family members or witnesses to dictate a treatment plan? Do they let weather affect whether the patient gets the standard of care? Environment? Workload? Sleep deprivation? Identify these factors if it is negatively influencing your candidate's decision-making process.

Risk vs. Reward. Does your candidate demonstrate an understanding of the risk and reward of certain interventions? Do they evaluate it, or just act rashly? Do they weigh risk vs. reward and then intervene accordingly?

Analyze and Anticipate. Does your candidate anticipate the expected outcome of interventions performed? Are they ready for side effects? Are they too worried and cautious so now they can't act? Do they overanalyze the situation? Paralysis by analysis?

4

Phase 1: Assimilation

Assimilation must be undertaken at the beginning of training. Whether this is a student doing an internship with a local paramedic school or a candidate for field instruction, this is the key to beginning an environment for success. The candidate must be allowed to assimilate into the team that you are currently working in, whether that is in a firehouse or on an ambulance crew. Assimilation is the vehicle that builds trust and confidence with your candidate.

The beginning of phase 1 starts with assimilation. There are two ways that the candidate must assimilate. First, they must assimilate into the team. Second, they must assimilate into their new role as a paramedic.

Assimilation into the team. Your candidate must feel warm and welcome with your crew. You must develop an atmosphere where they understand that they are there to learn how to operate as a paramedic. They are not there to serve you and your team. They are there to learn how to be a paramedic.

Assimilate your candidate into the team by including them in all of the activities that you and your crew routinely do. If your crew eats and cooks together, then they should be included. If your team cleans the station together, then they should be included. If your crew cleans the ambulance together, then they should be included. If your team goes out and trains together, then they should be included. And not only included, they must be integrated into the training and into the cleaning and into the eating.

Incorporating the student or candidate into these seemingly routine tasks is vitally important. What this does is silently starts to develop teamwork with your student and the rest of the crew. It develops communication and identifies how people function in relation to one another. Make no mistake—this will absolutely translate to the field, in a critical situation.

You should not act as if your candidate is just a student and put them in the corner and not allow them to be integrated into the team. This will cause lots of problems. Your candidate will never be able to act confidently because they are not confident that the team is behind them.

If your team is unmotivated and lacks the professionalism to include someone into their team, you must, as the preceptor, act as a barrier between your candidate and the team. This is extremely important. Your candidate must be allowed on scene to direct and delegate other members of the team without feeling consternation. The other members of the team must also put their egos aside in order to allow the student to delegate to them their vision for patient care. This is the reason that assimilation into the team is of the utmost importance. Your candidate will be leading your other team members throughout different scenarios and calls.

Being a paramedic is about leadership and delegation; it is not about regurgitating medical information. If they are not allowed, or comfortable enough, to practice and develop the skills needed to lead a team, it will greatly stunt the candidate's growth.

> **Assimilation into the new role.** This is the second way that your candidate must assimilate. They must recognize that they are now acting in a different capacity. This must be reinforced and needs to be addressed early on in their training.

Your candidate is no longer functioning as an EMT basic. The way that your candidate assimilates into their new role is by demonstrating commitment. They must be committed to providing high-quality patient care. They must be committed to studying and properly interpreting the medical guidelines and protocols. They must be committed to ongoing learning. They must be committed to critical thinking. They must be committed to receiving constructive criticism. They must be committed to showing up on time with a professional attitude and ready to work. They must be committed to your leadership and allowing you, the instructor, to guide and mold them into a new paramedic.

Another way that your candidate demonstrates assimilation into their new role is through conviction. They must demonstrate to you that they are committed to the paramedics' duty to act. This is a critical point. Paramedics must be convinced of the fact that we must intervene for people. If the candidate is committed to these obligations, it will be manifested through interventions performed on their patients. It will be manifested by your candidate providing good quality professional advice to people in bad situations. It will be manifested by their genuine need and want to help people.

Another principle that must be addressed, when it comes to assimilating into the new role as paramedic, is that your student is now formally entering into a leadership position. They must be informed that they are now entering into that position. Your candidate must be informed that there are now other responsibilities that they have to take on. They must be informed that they will be required to delegate tasks. They must take ownership and responsibility for the outcome of their patients. They must take accountability for the patient care that is provided. They have to be informed that while delegating tasks they should not be micromanaging their team.

Whatever the task may be, they must allow their team to implement and execute that task without impatient oversight. They must be informed that they are now responsible to make sure that their team is capable of providing good patient care and executing the tasks that they delegate to them.

We have addressed assimilation and the two ways it must happen. It should take approximately 100 to 150 hours for this to happen. Your candidate must be allowed to run calls for approximately this time frame in order to properly assimilate into the team. In our experience it takes this long to build and develop trust in the relationship so that your candidate can now feel as though they have the freedom to delegate properly.

During this 100- to 150-hour phase, your candidate needs to be allowed to demonstrate what their capabilities are. This is extremely important. You as the instructor must sit back and intervene as little as possible. It is our belief that your candidate must be allowed to jump in headfirst. This is especially true for students who only have approximately 500 hours of internship.

If during this initial 100 to 150 hours you recognize that your candidate needs lots of help, then begin to intervene and develop a plan to help them. If your candidate is demonstrating to you a lack of confidence and a lack of decisiveness, then begin with the small tasks. This is where you would implement simple teaching plans (to be addressed later).

Begin with minor interventions that your candidate must make the decision to conduct. An example of this is allowing them to decide when to give Zofran, or when to do a 12 lead, or when to start an IV. If your candidate cannot decide when to start an IV, they will never decide when to intubate. Allowing the candidate to make easier decisions will start to build the process needed for them to make more critical decisions in the future.

This is not about regurgitating the indications and contraindications of Zofran to you; it is about allowing your candidate to independently decide when to give a patient Zofran. This demonstrates to you, when properly done, an understanding of the contraindications and indications of Zofran. And this begins the verification process of your candidate's understanding of medical principles.

If your candidate needs excessive help with their decision-making process, begin here with the small decisions. This will quickly grow into their being able to run an entire call and execute an entire treatment plan for a patient. Because they build upon the confidence that they do understand prehospital medicine and that they can intervene correctly when needed.

The overarching theme of phase 1 is assimilation. However, a few steps must be completed within the first few days of training. Preferably the first day, so as not to waste time.

Step 1

The first item in phase one that must be addressed is expectations. And more specifically the expectations you as the instructor have for yourself. You have to identify what your expectations are of yourself before the internship even begins. What do you expect to gain from training someone else?

Having expectations for yourself is important because it gives you a personal investment in the internship itself. Creating expectations for yourself will cause you to be more accountable to yourself and the student. You, the instructor, need a personal investment in the success of the student and success of the internship or field instruction.

Then develop and articulate the expectations that you have for your student. Sit down and think about what expectations you're going to require of them. Here is a brief list of expectations that you can have of your student:

- You're going to expect that they are in uniform ready to go to work.
- You're going to expect that they go through the med-box every day.
- You're going to expect that they go through all the medical equipment every day.
- You're going to expect that they come to you with some sort of question for the day or questions that they need to address.
- You're going to expect that they will be involved in the decision-making on every single call. They must be allowed to make decisions independent of the instructor. This builds confidence.
- You're going to expect that they communicate to you any concerns they are having.
- You're going to expect them to execute treatment plans as they see fit.
- You're going to expect them to act, instead of ask for permission.

Then you have to develop the expectations that your student can have of you—moreover, what they can expect from you as their preceptor:

- They can expect that you will be there every day.
- They can expect that you will go through the medications with them.
- They can expect that you as their preceptor will begin to develop their decision-making process.
- They can expect that you as their preceptor will begin to develop a methodical approach toward patient care with them.
- They can expect that you will be evaluating their calls.
- They can expect that you will begin to address deficiencies within their practice.
- They should also be able to expect that you will be fair.
- They can expect that you will give them liberty to make decisions without unnecessary punitive repercussions.
- They can expect that you are personally invested in the internship or field training.
- They can expect that you will not undermine their treatment unless it is for safety reasons or a lack in the standard of care.

Last, you, the instructor, have to allow the student to have the opportunity to voice their expectations of the internship and of you. Don't minimize the importance of allowing the student or the trainee to tell you what their expectations are. They will have expectations, and they should have expectations. This is their opportunity to tell you what they expect from you and what they expect from the field training. Keep in mind you might need to allow adequate time for the student to develop their thoughts and expectations.

Expectations must be addressed on day one. The candidate must know what is expected of them so that they can start to incorporate them into the internship. It is not acceptable to hold someone accountable for something that they do not know is expected of them. If your candidate is not doing something that you want them to, they may not know that you are expecting them to do it. Always look at yourself first and ensure that you have communicated to the candidate what you expect.

After the expectations are set, everybody begins with a clean slate and on the same page. Now there are no question marks as to what is expected.

Expectations

Expectations are important. Writing them down and articulating them forces you to keep yourself accountable. Revisit the expectations periodically to ensure that they are being met and to add to them if needed.

Expectations for yourself:

1. Learn something from my student.
2. Identify something deficient in my own practice.
3.
4.

Expectations you have for your student:

1. Be actively involved in decision-making on scene.
2. Show up on time ready to learn.
3. Listen to instruction and incorporate criticism into practice.
4.
5.
6.

What your student can expect from you:

1. Delegate responsibility for patient care to the student.
2. Provide constructive criticism.
3. Give positive and negative feedback.
4.
5.

What are the expectations your student has of you and the field instruction?

1. Be committed to the student's success.
2.
3.
4.
5.

Notes:

Step 2

Next: begin the evaluation process. What does the evaluation process look like and what does it entail? Where do you begin the evaluation process?

The evaluation process should begin after you formally give the candidate your expectations, which is why expectations should be given immediately. Allow your students some liberty to run a few alarms, take a few calls, and do a few assessments so that you can evaluate what they need to work on. Then you can begin to make teaching plans and then execute those plans.

When we talk about evaluation, you're evaluating their ability to run an alarm and make good decisions. Here are a few key attributes and characteristics that you have to continually evaluate in order to determine whether or not they're proficient and capable of functioning independently:

- You have to evaluate their basic understanding or knowledge of medical principles. This is verification.
- You have to evaluate the application of that knowledge. This will consume most of your time with the internship—evaluating their ability to apply what they know.
- You have to evaluate their communication abilities. Communication is key to being a paramedic, and you must evaluate how effective they are at it.
- You have to evaluate their ability to work within a team. You have to evaluate whether or not they can function as a team member and also a team leader.
- You have to evaluate their ability to delegate tasks. They have to apply the knowledge that they've got, but they also have to be able to delegate tasks to other team members. This is essential for a successful paramedic.

- You have to evaluate their skills. Are they competent and capable of performing skills? For example can they start IVs? Can they intubate? Can they perform a physical exam? These are skills that must be evaluated by you, the preceptor.
- When it comes to evaluations, the decision-making process is what you're evaluating. You have to evaluate whether or not the student is sure of themselves. Are they confident? Are they assertive? Do they hesitate? Do they make bad decisions? Do they make decisions based on emotion rather than on objective information?
- Finally, you as a preceptor must continually evaluate the candidate's professionalism.

Evaluation Forms

The following evaluations should be done at 50- to 100-hour increments during your training of the student. It allows you to make adjustments, as needed, and assure that you are making progress with your candidate.

Student/Candidate Self-Evaluation

Have the candidate evaluate themselves on a 1–10 scale for each of the following categories:

1 is the lowest confidence in themselves

10 is the highest confidence in themselves

Do this self-evaluation at the beginning of training and at the end of training.

- Communication
- Teamwork
- Leadership
- Patient Assessment
- Delegation
- Setting the Tone
- Decision-Making
- General Medical Knowledge
- Application of Knowledge
- Methods of Action

- Flexibility in Treatment Plans
- Assertiveness
- Confidence

On the following evaluation forms, use the scale 1 to 5:

1 Candidate does not demonstrate the knowledge required to make informed decisions about a patient's treatment plans. If scores of 1 are demonstrated, it is incumbent upon the student to take the necessary measures to inform their intellect to a level at which they can now make decisions. This is a critical moment. Will they invest in themselves the work needed to learn medicine?

3 Candidate meets the bare minimum of understanding to create and implement treatment plans. Candidate still requires prompting on most calls. Able to function on BLS calls but still has difficulty with complex ALS calls.

5 Candidate exceeds the knowledge that is required of them and has a very good grasp of medical principles needed to operate independently as a paramedic. This is demonstrated by the candidate routinely implementing the correct treatment plans independently from instructor input.

Medical Principles

Does your student demonstrate proficiency in the following disciplines?

Cardiology				
1	2	3	4	5

Pharmacology

1 2 3 4 5

Anatomy/Physiology

1 2 3 4 5

Pulmonology

1 2 3 4 5

Altered Mental Status

1 2 3 4 5

Infections

1 2 3 4 5

Guidelines or Protocols

1 2 3 4 5

Trauma

1 2 3 4 5

Airway Management and Anatomy

1 2 3 4 5

OB Emergencies

1 2 3 4 5

Pediatric

1 2 3 4 5

CVA

1 2 3 4 5

Capnography

1 2 3 4 5

Any other medical knowledge you deem applicable and necessary as the instructor.

________________ 1 2 3 4 5

________________ 1 2 3 4 5

________________ 1 2 3 4 5

During your evaluation if you find 3s and below, use these scores to identify an area that should be addressed. The goal is to have a minimum of 3s, which would be identified as average, in every discipline.

- What areas need to be addressed?
- What is your plan to help your student improve upon these areas? Write it down and include the student in developing a teaching plan.
- What is today's date? This will hold you more accountable and give you a tool to measure success.

Interpersonal Skills

Does your student demonstrate the interpersonal skills necessary to be a successful paramedic (score from 1 to 5)?

1 Candidate does not demonstrate the ability of the associated skill set. Needs constant prompting or guidance.

3 Candidate is able to effectively implement treatment plans on BLS calls but still has difficulty on complex ALS calls.

5 Candidate routinely demonstrates the associated skill set with no prompting from the instructor. The candidate is easily able to navigate any call that is in front of them from start to finish.

Communication

1 **2** **3** **4** **5**

Teamwork

1 **2** **3** **4** **5**

Leadership

1	2	3	4	5

Patient Assessment

1	2	3	4	5

Delegation

1	2	3	4	5

Setting the Tone

1	2	3	4	5

Decision-Making

1	2	3	4	5

During your evaluation if you find 3s and below, you need to identify and address this area with your student. The goal is to have at minimum a 3, which would be identified as average, in every discipline.

- What areas need to be addressed?
- What is your teaching plan to improve upon these areas? Write it down and include the student in developing a teaching plan.
- What is today's date? This will hold you more accountable and give you a tool to measure success.

Tools to Improve Skills

These tools are just a brief starting point. If you have methods that work already, then implement those tools. Make sure you identify for yourself clearly what it is that you are teaching or trying to improve by using your own tools.

Communication

Give your student pictures to look at for 30 seconds and then ask them to communicate effectively to you what is in the picture in 45 seconds or less.

Have your student give a class on capnography and evaluate whether they are communicating the information appropriately.

Record your student giving practice hand-off reports to other agencies or the hospital so they can hear what they sound like.

Teamwork

Your student must run the calls, all of them. To some degree they must be involved in the decision-making on every single call you run. They must work within the team to implement their vision for patient care. Force them to make decisions and delegate tasks.

Leadership

Run scenarios and have your student take the lead within your crew. This will build confidence, teamwork, communication, and delegation. Allow your student to run the call with absolutely zero input from you, the instructor. Do allow for team members to voice their opinions as if it is a real call.

Have your student come up with a training calendar for the day and allow them the opportunity and latitude to implement it as they see fit.

Patient Assessment

Reflect on the line of questioning on each call you go on with your student. Why did they ask what they asked? What information were they trying to get and why? Did they get the information? Was it pertinent? Did they implement a good treatment plan based on that information? Did they correctly interpret the information that they gathered?

Delegation

Have the student practice giving tasks to other team members. Don't allow the student to perform all of the interventions or, in some cases, any.

Setting the Tone (Tones 3 Cs)

Command: Do they take command of the call or are they timid?

Conviction: Do they demonstrate the conviction to act. Do they understand duty to act, implied consent? Are they convinced that as paramedics they must intervene for people?

Confident: Do they communicate the plan confidently to team members? Or are they easily swayed and unable to make a decision?

Your student must run the calls. They cannot learn to make decisions by watching you make decisions. Once your student becomes comfortable in the learning environment you create and understands that they will not be told what to do, and have liberty to do as they see fit, they will grow exponentially. Obviously, intervene if necessary to maintain the standard of care for your patient. Do not willingly allow for negligent care to be conducted by your student.

Qualities to Evaluate and Develop within Your Candidate

Humility. Is your student humble? To give you more clarity on what humility looks like, ask yourself this. Does your student respond well to constructive criticism? Do they take your direction and mentorship well or are they making excuses and interjecting instead of following your lead? To determine if the student is being humble, you must be actively engaged in mentoring them. This does not include showing them how awesome you are. Mentoring them does not include telling your student about all the cool calls you have run. They don't care. If a call is not applicable to the mentorship, then don't discuss it. Here is the key, humility in your student starts with humility in you as the instructor.

Ego/Pride. Is your student prideful and arrogant? Obviously this is the antithesis to humility. Is the student making rash decisions in arrogance? Do they know everything all the time? Do they disregard your input and mentorship? This quality must be addressed, however, and once again this starts with you as the instructor. Are you prideful and arrogant? Here is a little insight—nobody cares how awesome you think you are, or how many calls you run. It is absolutely fruitless to demonstrate this to your student. Learning is hindered. Do you know why it is hindered? Because your arrogance demonstrates to your student that you are precepting them to your benefit and exultation; you are not doing it for your student's benefit. Your student recognizes this. Your student will respond much better if you start by checking your own ego first.

Compassion. Is your student compassionate with others? The primary focus here is the patient. There may be certain situations or patients that trigger your student to become frustrated and upset. This is okay, and it is realistic. What is important, however, is to recognize such situations so that you can address it. When your student knows more clearly how they react to certain situations, it will improve their patient care.

Empathy. Is your student empathetic? Do they treat patients with a judgmental attitude? Understand that sometimes people become frustrated and overwhelmed with certain patients, which is okay, but the overarching attitude shouldn't exhibit hate and judgment. They will be better at treating patients if they are able to understand where people are coming from and be empathetic to it.

Accountability. Does your student hold themselves accountable for their actions and interventions? Again, this starts with you as the instructor. Do you hold them accountable for the expectations that you have discussed?

Responsibility. This goes hand-in-hand with accountability. Does your student take responsibility for their actions? Do they take responsibility for treatment plans they implement? This is key. If your student is not willing to own the treatment that they implement, they will never be able to act decisively. Acting decisively is about owning what you do. It's not about understanding every nuance of medicine.

Passion. What drives your student? Help your student develop a good understanding of why they became a paramedic in the first place. Of course this always begins with a desire to help others. But why do they want to help others? That is the real question that needs to be answered. When that question is answered and articulated clearly in the mind of your student, it will drive them toward excellence. Help them develop this answer and understand the importance of it.

Integrity. This one is simple. Does your student exhibit integrity? This is demonstrated every day by working with you as the instructor. Do they try to get out of work? Are they lying to you about anything? Do they do what is right when you are not there? Are you able to give them an assignment with confidence they will follow through and accomplish it? A lack in integrity is demonstrated by making excuses and blaming others for poor outcomes instead of taking responsibility for those outcomes. Your student's lack of integrity will affect patient care, and they will blame others for things when they shouldn't.

Assessment of Qualities

1 Candidate does not demonstrate the associated attribute, so extensive counseling is needed by the instructor. If your candidate demonstrates a score of 1 in these areas, it may be cause for major concern. These qualities should be present even at the beginning of training.

3 Candidate demonstrates an ability to interact with patients and teammates well enough to navigate a call. A score of 3 demonstrates there is still room for improvement with bedside manner and self-discipline.

5 Candidate demonstrates routinely an ability to connect with your patients and team, and seamlessly executes an appropriate treatment plan. Your candidate is routinely able to accept constructive criticism and learn from it by implementing your feedback quickly into their mode of treating patients. Your candidate routinely demonstrates a willingness to take accountability for their actions and makes no excuses for decisions made.

Qualities: Identify and evaluate these qualities in your student. Under *passion* realize that this is something for which you should help your student come to understand for themselves. As the mentor and instructor, you need to address these qualities if your student needs it.Again these look so great.

Humility

1	2	3	4	5

Ego/Pride

1	2	3	4	5

Compassion

1	2	3	4	5

Empathy

1 2 3 4 5

Accountability

1 2 3 4 5

Responsibility

1 2 3 4 5

Passion

1 2 3 4 5

Integrity

1 2 3 4 5

Skills Evaluation

1 Candidate cannot perform the skill, does not demonstrate an ability to successfully perform the skill or understand when to implement the intervention.

3 Candidate performs the skill adequately enough to provide patient care. Improvement and practice still needed to be proficient and work independently. Is still hesitant, unsure of themselves, and fails 50 percent of the time.

5 Candidate routinely performs the skill with no instructions from the evaluator.

Intubation

1	2	3	4	5

IV

1	2	3	4	5

12 lead Placement

1	2	3	4	5

12 lead Interpretation

1	2	3	4	5

Patient Assessment

1	2	3	4	5

Capnography Interpretation

1	2	3	4	5

Bleeding Control

1	2	3	4	5

Cardiac Monitor Usage

1 2 3 4 5

Medication Administration

1 2 3 4 5

Step 3

Now you've done your initial evaluation. You have given the candidate liberty to demonstrate their capabilities, and you should have identified what they need to work on. The initial evaluation is extremely important because it gives you the opportunity as the preceptor to identify deficiencies with your student.

The next step is to develop teaching plans. Teaching plans can be simple or complex. Keep in mind that you have to develop a teaching plan with your student's input. The student needs to have buy-in on the plan and also a clear understanding of what the objectives are set forth in the plan. They know what their goals are and what is to be done in order to meet those goals.

The teaching plan can be simple in terms of studying cardiology for fifteen minutes a day because you have identified that they are deficient in their ability to read 12 leads. That is a simple teaching plan. A complex teaching plan develops the candidate's ability to function more completely. It incorporates multiple aspects of successfully running a call, such as skills and delegation.

What goes into the teaching plan? Simple. Begin with the overall objective. Then within that objective, decide what goals must be met in order to successfully reach the objective. For example, does the student need to work on communication skills, delegation, differential diagnosis, or their line of questioning?

What are the benchmarks within each goal that have to be met in order to reach the goal? For example, they have to meet the benchmark of coming up with five differentials per patient, or successfully assessing a patient without interrupting the patient. Or successfully delegating a task to a team member. The benchmarks are set forth within the goals, and the goals are set forth within the objective.

Teaching Plans

Date:

Complex Teaching Plan

A complex teaching plan involves several steps.

- Plan objective
- Goals to meet the objective
- Benchmarks to meet the goals

Complex Teaching Plan Objective

Goals to Meet the Teaching Plan Objective

1.
2.
3.

Benchmarks to Meet the Goals

Objective Goal number 1

Benchmark 1:

Benchmark 2:

Objective Goal number 2

Benchmark 1:

Benchmark 2:

Objective Goal number 3

Benchmark 1:

Benchmark 2:

This is a complex teaching plan outline, but this should not become cumbersome and difficult. Develop the plan with your student and then execute and reevaluate.

Example-Teaching Plan

Date:

Complex Teaching Plan Example

A complex teaching plan involves several steps:

- Plan objective
- Goals to meet the objective
- Benchmarks to meet the goals

Complex Teaching Plan Objective: *Build confidence with student in their decision-making and execution*

Goals to Meet the Teaching Plan Objective:

1. *Identify which stage of the decision-making process the student is having difficulty with. Example: Interpretation? Categorizing? Prioritizing? Execution?*
2. *Have student create and present a class on any discipline they feel they need to understand better. Example: Capnography, EKGs, cardiology, respiratory, OB*
3. *Implement team-building exercises and activities.*

Benchmarks to Meet the Goals

Objective Goal Number 1

1. Benchmark 1: *Candidate is able to define each stage and how it relates to ten consecutive patients that they interact with.*
2. Benchmark 2: *Candidate is able to verbalize on scene why each intervention is performed, correctly and confidently.*

Objective Goal Number 2

1. Benchmark 1: *Candidate gives a class on capnography (or whatever the candidate chooses) and demonstrates proficiency with understanding of V/Q mismatch, waveform and End Tidal CO2*
2. Benchmark 2: *Candidate properly identified the next five patients that needed capnography and correctly interpreted the findings.*

Objective Goal Number 3

1. Benchmark 1: *Candidate successfully delegates tasks to teammates in five scenarios.*
2. Benchmark 2: *Candidate successfully learns three things about each teammate that is unrelated to the Fire Service or EMS, while at the same time providing each member with three things about themselves that is unrelated to the Fire Service or EMS.*

Date:

Complex Teaching Plan Evaluation

1 Does not meet objective

3 Minimum standard for objective met

5 Exceeds standard for objective

Overall Objective

1 2 3 4 5

Goal number 1

1 2 3 4 5

Benchmark 1

1 2 3 4 5

Benchmark 2

1 2 3 4 5

Goal number 2

1 2 3 4 5

Benchmark 1

1 2 3 4 5

Benchmark 2

1 2 3 4 5

Goal number 3

1 2 3 4 5

Benchmark 1

1 2 3 4 5

Benchmark 2

1 2 3 4 5

Notes:

The complex teaching plan should only be implemented one objective at a time. With a score of 3 or lower, you are advised to continue to execute the plan or change the execution. A score of 4 and above demonstrates competence, so move on to other areas that need improvement.

Date:

Simple Teaching Plan

Remember, your simple teaching plan is just that: simple. This should be very specific (for example, give three differentials on every call, or start an IV, or read an EKG properly). Don't allow the simple plan to become global and large in scope; that is for the complex plan.

Simple Plan Objective

Plan of Execution

1	2	3	4	5

Plan Evaluation

1	2	3	4	5

Notes:

This is a simple teaching plan. Develop the plan with your student. Form a plan of execution and then execute and evaluate. Keep in mind, multiple simple teaching plans can be in play simultaneously. Do not implement multiple complex teaching plans simultaneously. With a score of 3 or lower, you are advised to continue to execute the plan or change the execution. A score of 4 and above demonstrates competence, so move on to other areas that need improvement.

Date:

Simple Teaching Plan—Example

Remember, your simple teaching plan is just that: simple. This should be very specific (for example, give three differentials on every call, or start an IV, or read an EKG properly). Don't allow the simple plan to become global and large in scope; that is for the complex plan.

Simple Plan Objective

Become more accurate with reading 12 lead EKGs

Plan of Execution

Read cardiology for twenty minutes each shift and work through an EKG workbook.

Plan Evaluation

1 2 3 4 5

Notes:

Step 4

After you've developed your teaching plans based on your evaluations, the next logical step is to implement the teaching plan. You must hold yourself to that plan. Go out the door and execute the teaching plan that you have set forth with your student.

What comes next is the evaluation of the plan. You have to evaluate whether the plan worked or whether it didn't work. Then you are able to tweak the teaching plan here and there to see what will be more effective. Maybe on the next call you change one little part of the teaching plan so that you can better evaluate it or you can implement it.

This concludes everything that should be accomplished in phase 1 during the 100 to 150 hours needed to properly assimilate your student into the team and into the new role. It also takes this long for you to develop trust with your candidate that you won't undermine the treatment that they are implementing.

At the end of this phase the candidate should have the utmost confidence to say to you, "I'm giving some fentanyl, will you go get it out of the rig?" If your reply is "Yes, sir" or "Yes, ma'am," then you have successfully created the environment and assimilation of phase 1.

5

Phase 2: Verification, Decision-Making, Leadership Development

Phase 2 of the field training will pick up right on the heels of phase 1. Phase 2 is easily the most labor intensive for you as the instructor. Three primary tasks that must be addressed within phase 2 are verification, decision-making and the development of methodical approaches, and leadership development.

Verification

Specifically what skills are you as the instructor trying to verify in your trainee? The goal here is to verify medical principles and the understanding of clinical knowledge. You have to ensure that the paramedics that you are training have a high degree of proficiency with understanding medical knowledge.

Verification begins in phase 1 during the student's assimilation. You can begin verifying the candidate's understanding of medical principles while they are implementing treatment plans, and begin to address skills you deem necessary.

Phase 2, however, should be devoted to making sure that your student understands the medical principles needed to operate as an independent paramedic. This does not mean that you play *Jeopardy!* with your student and ask them to parrot back information that they learned in a textbook. The way to properly verify the information that they know is to allow them to run calls and then ask them questions post call about the interventions they performed.

Here's an example: If a patient receives albuterol treatments, then after the call you ask about these related issues:

- COPD
- Reactive airway disease
- Albuterol treatments
- Atrovent treatments
- Corticosteroids
- Magnesium
- Epinephrine
- Breathing treatments
- CPAP
- Emergent returns versus nonemergent returns
- When and how to manage a patient's airway
- The proper breathing rates for people
- The signs of a difficulty breathing patient

You take the time at this point, after running the call, to go over in depth and verify the student's understanding. After a call, the student has a context for that information. They're not just repeating something they've learned in a classroom; they're putting that learning in the context with a call that they just ran. This allows the student to see firsthand the application of their medical knowledge.

By going over critical information at this point, you start to develop a methodical approach for each individual candidate. The candidate, unbeknownst to them, is starting to create their own methods by which to intervene when presented with a patient's complaint, illness, or injury. If you allow them the latitude to implement treatment plans as they see fit—and then demonstrate to you understanding of why they did those things after the fact—they will start to create their own methods.

When you verify in this manor, you create an enormous amount of confidence within the student, because they are not solely relying on your input for treatment plans. Their growth starts to develop exponentially.

The most difficult part of phase 2 ironically is that the instructor needs to just stay out of the way. Allow the student to develop and execute treatment plans as they see fit within local protocols and guidelines. If you verify your candidate's knowledge after the fact, you are reinforcing to your student or candidate that they do know when to properly implement certain interventions.

This approach reinforces that they do understand indications and contraindications of medications. Then the next time they see a similar situation, they're more likely to have the confidence to implement and execute treatment plans that are needed for the patient in front of them. Your candidate is no longer starting at square one because you've gone over with them in context and reinforced their understanding of medical principles and how they are to be applied to patients. Your candidate now begins to slowly work independently of you, the instructor.

Here is a list of specifics that need to be verified that follow the standard as set forth by your medical directors.

1. Cardiology
    a. ACS
    b. STEMI
    c. ACLS
    d. Pulmonary Embolism
    e. DVTs and Arterial Blocks
2. Pharmacology
    a. Indications
    b. Contraindications
    c. Dosages
    d. 6 Rights
3. Respiratory Diseases and Treatments
    a. COPD
    b. CHF
    c. Asthma
    d. Pneumonia
    e. Choking
    f. Croup
    g. Epiglottitis
4. Basic Anatomy and Physiology
    a. Heart

   b. Lungs
   c. Acid Base
   d. Kidney Failure
   e. Endocrine and Diabetic Emergency
5. Altered Mental Status
   a. Intoxicated Party
   b. Overdose
   c. Seizure
   d. Any Altered Patient
6. Infections
   a. Sepsis
7. Guidelines and Protocols (such as)
   a. Destination Guidelines
   b. DOA
   c. Refusals
   d. Standing Orders
   e. Triage
8. Allergic Reactions
   a. Anaphylaxis
9. Trauma
   a. Bleeding Control
   b. Tension Pneumothorax
   c. Multisystems Trauma
   d. Cushings Triad

10. Airway Management and Anatomy
    a. Intubation
    b. RSI (if applicable)
    c. Cricothyrotomy
    d. Supraglottic Airway Device
    e. BLS Skills
    f. **Note here that aggressive management of the airway is critical in prehospital medicine and must be addressed.**
11. OB Emergencies
    a. Imminent Delivery
    b. Breech Delivery
    c. Prolapsed Cord
    d. Eclampsia/Pre-eclampsia
12. Pediatric
    a. Destination Hospitals
    b. Broselow Tape or Similar Devices
    c. Pediatric Pharmacology
13. CVA
    a. Ischemic
    b. Hemorrhagic
    c. Identification (Cincinnati prehospital stroke scale)
    d. Destination Hospitals
14. Capnography
    a. ETCO2

   b. Waveform
   c. V/Q Mismatch
   d. ETT Confirmation (if applicable)

Clinical knowledge is not the only skill that must be verified and developed. Here is a list of attributes that must also be verified and developed.

1. Communication Skills
   a. With Patients
   b. With Teammates
   c. With Other Agencies
   d. With Hospital
2. Teamwork
   a. With Team
   b. With Other Agencies
3. Leadership
   a. Setting the Tone
      i. Command
      ii. Conviction
      iii. Confidence
   b. Delegation
   c. Implementation of Vision
   d. Does Not Micromanage
   e. Ownership and Accountability
   f. Professionalism

Decision-Making

Developing your candidate's decision-making process is going to take the vast majority of your time. Decision-making was laid out earlier in the book, so please refer back to that section.

Understand that creating a paramedic who can make sound decisions is only possible by forcing the individual to actually make decisions independent from your input. **Your candidate cannot learn how to make decisions by watching you make decisions**. In order to make good decisions, the candidate must be forced to make decisions on every single call. And then after the call is over, this is where general and self-reflection comes into play.

Every single call should be evaluated and discussed why the decisions were made and what the candidate saw that caused them to make the decision that they did make. This reinforces why they're making certain decisions and reinforces their ability to interpret information correctly.

Through the decision-making process, we are attempting to develop four principles within each candidate:

- Step one is interpreting information.
- Step two is categorizing information.
- Step three is prioritizing treatment plans.
- Step four is execution of the treatment plan.

Defining decision-making in this way helps the candidate understand what it is that you are looking for as the instructor. Defining decision-making in this manner with four specific goals in mind gives them a clear indicator for how to make decisions. Implementing and defining these four principles for each candidate gives you the ability to break down their decision-making process and more accurately identify hesitations in making decisions.

Using these four steps of decision-making as a template for your student to build upon will reduce hesitation in the field.

1. This approach allows you to verify whether or not they can correctly interpret their understanding of clinical information. Do they correctly interpret the clinical findings present in each patient that they go on?
2. Second, this approach verifies whether or not the student is able to categorize the information that they are interpreting correctly (for example, is it a respiratory call, a cardiac call, a traumatic injury, and so on?).
3. Next, you are able to evaluate the prioritizing of treatment plans. Does your candidate demonstrate the ability to understand when to implement the interventions needed for each specific patient? And are they able to prioritize those actions so that the most important steps get done first? Airway, for example, comes before everything else.
4. The last principle here of execution allows you to verify your candidate's ability to lead a team through a call. This tests the candidate's leadership and communication abilities, which are critical in paramedicine. This also evaluates whether the student actively engages or hesitates.

Reflecting on these four principles is where your student's decision-making process gets built.

Execution should be defined in this way: vision. Is your candidate able to create a vision for a treatment plan for each patient and then properly delegate and lead the team through it? They must develop a vision for how to treat each patient.

After developing the vision, how are they going to implement it? Vision, however, does not stop with just the treatment plan.

What is the vision for getting the patient out of the house? Or extricating them from the vehicle? Do you need a truck company or other help? Does the patient need a stair chair? Are you going back to the hospital emergent? Is it a refusal? In short, what the student must develop is an overall vision for how the call is going to be run from start to finish, and then execute it through teamwork. This is what you are evaluating and developing.

Here is an example of what this looks like. You get a call for a shortness of breath patient. Upon arrival your candidate begins to question the patient about their difficulty breathing. Your candidate listens to their lung sounds and recognizes wheezing. Stop. This is exactly what we are looking for. Before you go any further, is your candidate able to recognize the shortness of breath, recognize that they need to listen to lung sounds, and then recognize the wheezing? And then are they able to correctly interpret the wheezing and how to address it?

Are they able to categorize this patient as a difficulty breathing patient or reactive airway disease patient? Does your candidate understand that this patient is a respiratory patient? Next, are they able to prioritize a treatment plan? Do they understand that they need to perform certain interventions before other interventions?

Depending on how sick the respiratory patient is dictates what interventions need to be done first. Is this a patient who needs epinephrine first? Is this a patient that simply needs an albuterol treatment first? This is where you must force your student to make the decision for what their treatment plan is going to be. They must prioritize the interventions needed.

Once they have prioritized the interventions, are they able to execute their vision for patient care through communication and delegation? Do they have the confidence and ability to delegate tasks to other team members? Are they able to ask others to quickly and definitively start an albuterol treatment? Are they able to quickly and definitively ask others to get oxygen, or to get a set of vitals? Summed up in this example is vision: Is the student able to implement their vision?

When it comes to decision-making, practice builds confidence. Do not allow your candidate the pleasure of informing them what you would do on a call; require them to decide what to do. If needed, start with small things, like deciding who a patient is, or when to do vital signs or start IVs. Then move to bigger or more difficult decisions.

The candidate must practice the art of delegation and direction. They must practice directing teammates to start interventions.

Now this must be stated again: If you need to intervene, then intervene, but this should be the exception not the rule. If you are intervening on every call, then something is wrong. What is wrong the vast majority of time is instructor ego, because you won't allow the candidate to do it their way. If it is a problem with the candidate, then back up and start with small things. Then build from there. Some candidates can take a year to develop, but if their mentality is right, you should be able to make them successful.

For more information on decision-making, refer to our book *Life and Death Matters: Professionalism and Decision-Making for the First Responder.* In this book is a section devoted to many factors that affect decision-making. Understanding these factors and identifying them will greatly improve your ability to help others develop a good decision-making process.

Leadership

Leadership goes hand-in-hand with decision-making. Some of the factors that will directly impact leadership capabilities are communication skills, delegation skills, accountability, ownership, and, maybe most importantly, conviction.

If you, as a paramedic, are committed to the responsibilities in front of you, it will make you more decisive. Accountability equals liberty. If you take accountability for the decisions you make, it directly affects your ability to make decisions. This notion must be instilled into your student or candidate.

In phase 2 your candidate's leadership skills must be addressed and then developed if need be. The two skills that are most critical are communication and delegation. In order to develop these skills, you must allow your candidate to actively use them. They must be thrust into the environment of having to create a vision for a treatment plan and then communicate that vision and delegate tasks to teammates. These skills need to be specifically addressed and developed.

You cannot simply discuss these skills; they must be practiced and utilized on scene by the candidate, because that is how they develop them. It is important that you allow the candidate latitude to navigate this new role on their own and develop their own way of communicating to people. Do not force them to do everything the way that you do it; otherwise, the process won't be natural to them.

These seven items must be addressed, defined, and developed within your candidate as it relates to leadership:

- Leader's intent
- Delegation
- Ownership
- Commitment
- Setting the tone
- Micromanagement
- Gray situations

What is **leader's intent** and how does that relate to the paramedic? Leader's intent is a statement that defines what team members must know in order to be successful for a given objective. This intent will outline three basic concepts.

As it relates to the paramedic, leader's intent must be developed within your team prior to going on a call. Leader's intent within EMS is a more global picture of patient care in general and does not relate specifically to any individual patient or a specific call. The first concept developed within leader's intent is the objective. What is the objective of the paramedic and what is the objective of the paramedic's team? The objective for us here is *to provide the highest quality standard of patient care* that we can possibly provide on every single call. That is the objective.

The second concept here is the *reason*. In order for the team to function properly, function at a high degree of proficiency, and function independently of the paramedic, they must understand why. Your team (and your student is part of that team) must understand why you have the objective of providing the highest quality patient care. The why is that we as paramedics are obligated and committed to advocate for our patients in every single circumstance we see. The why is that we must be committed to our duty to act and know that we need to advocate for our patients. That is the why. And it is your job as preceptor to convey that reason to your student.

The third concept here to be developed is *success*. What does a successful outcome look like? What is the end result that we are looking for? The end result that we are trying to achieve is consistent and reliable patient care. This is demonstrated by providing high-quality patient care on every single call, which is demonstrated by having a true compassion for your patient and advocating for their best interest. This is how you know that you have successfully defined your intention for your team. The word that we use for individual calls is *vision*. Vision is the leader's intent for the individual call. This concept must be developed within your candidate.

The next principle here that needs to be developed is **delegation**. Delegation can be rather simple. You must allow your candidate to delegate tasks. If this is something that your candidate has difficulty with, then you need to practice this at the station or in the back of your ambulance with your team. You can do this by running scenarios in order to make them more comfortable with delegating tasks.

Practicing the art of delegation can take a lot of time and reinforcement on the part of the instructor. Remember that you need to give both positive and negative feedback to the candidate. Understand that the idea of delegation is integrated within leader's intent. **Delegation is the vehicle by which the leader is capable of accomplishing their vision.**

The next concept is **ownership**. You must instill a sense of ownership within your candidate. They must take accountability for their actions. When your candidate takes accountability for their actions, it demonstrates to you that they have an understanding of the consequences of their actions. This must be demonstrated throughout the entire internship or field instruction process. Ownership has to be demonstrated on calls, not just talked about. This is extremely important.

If someone is not willing to take accountability and own the decisions that they make, it will hinder their ability to make good decisions and may prevent them from being decisive in critical situations. This is at the essence of the so-called gray situation, which is discussed shortly.

The next concept is **commitment**. The candidate must display a level of commitment to the role of paramedic. They must be committed to the fact that they have a new role. They must be committed to the fact that they are now in a leadership position. They must be committed to providing high-quality patient care. They must be committed to proper preparation in order to provide that good quality patient care. They must be committed to keeping up on all of the knowledge that is required of them. And they must be committed to be a patient advocate first and always. This is something that needs to be formally addressed.

The next concept is **setting the tone**. Setting the tone is defined with the "Tone's 3 Cs": *Command*: your student needs to develop a command presence. This is developed and demonstrated by your student's willingly asserting themselves into a leadership position. This does not mean you should train your student to bark orders at the team. Delegation can be done subtly; it is less effective if your candidate is aggressive. The largest beneficiary of command, however, is the patient. The patient can immediately recognize that someone is actively in charge and taking the responsibility to mitigate their emergency. This will absolutely help your student develop consistent patient rapport.

Conviction: your candidate must be committed to the fact that they have a duty to act. This conviction will in turn provide them with the tools for leading people through a critical situation. Conviction incorporated with accountability will give your candidate the ability to act decisively in critical situations. The student must be committed to the fact they must advocate for their patient.

Confidence: this is the third C. Leading with confidence is key. Making decisions with confidence must be instilled into your student. How do you as the instructor develop confidence in your student? Preparation and accountability. Help your student prepare for situations, such as developing methodical approaches to patient care. Then taking accountability for the decisions made are the tools that will build confidence for your student. Setting the proper tone is critical to effective leadership. The Tone's 3 Cs defines how to do it.

Let's address **micromanagement**. Micromanagement in general demonstrates the intent of the leader as undefined and goes hand-in-hand with poor leadership. It also demonstrates a lack of trust in the team. If you have properly created an environment in which your team understands what the leader's intent is, your candidate will be able to function independently of your input. If you micromanage your candidate, you will in turn teach them to micromanage their teams, which will in turn cause patient care to suffer.

Micromanagement is at the heart of arrogance and can lead to poor patient care and poor patient advocacy. The student must be informed that they need to allow their teammates to perform tasks and interventions independently. Nobody likes to be micromanaged, and micromanagement is a sign of poor leadership. If your team is not capable of performing simple tasks and interventions that are asked of them, it is a direct reflection of your lack of leadership, lack of proper preparation, and lack of communicating your intent as a leader.

This leads to the last concept that needs to be addressed—the ever infectious **gray situation**. Gray situations do not exist. Do not infect your candidate with the belief that they are not capable of solving problems because the situation may seem convoluted. The sheer fact that we go on so many different calls with so many different variables with so many difficult decisions to make reinforces the fact that we must be decisive and take accountability for actions. We cannot chalk it up to an excuse of a gray situation.

Reinforce this with your candidate, and your candidate will be better off. They will act more decisively, more definitively, and take more accountability for their actions, and in turn provide much higher quality patient care because now the decisions take on a personal reflection. These decisions are now understood to have purpose and meaning, which directly impacts patient care. They are not making decisions in haste or with little consideration because they are inconsequential given the gray situation. Having this mentality is crucial because, in the end, it causes individuals to become better and better.

Don't allow the candidate to use a so-called gray situation as an excuse for indecision. Require them to be decisive and then own the decision. This by default forces preparation for those difficult situations, and they will ultimately provide better patient care. **Demanding that paramedics be decisive leaders, then in the same breath allow for gray situations to permeate treatment plans is counterintuitive.**

Addressing these seven concepts formally and routinely within the field instruction program will reinforce to your candidate that they can and will make good decisions. And that they have the tools by which to make those good decisions. It reinforces to your candidate that you are interested in their leadership abilities and their ability to advocate for your patient rather than just in their ability to interpret a 12 lead.

Your candidate can now have confidence that they can go out the door and meet the various challenges that they will face. Reinforcing these concepts during the field instruction process will show your candidate that they do have the capability of working independently of your instruction and oversight.

Phase 2 is also extremely important to build the candidate's confidence. After discussing and evaluating these principles set forth, the candidate understands that you as the preceptor are not simply requiring them to regurgitate information, or mimic you as a provider. They begin to understand that you as a preceptor are concerned with mentoring and developing them as a complete provider.

Phase 2 is by far the most extensive phase. This concludes after the candidate has shown proficiency in all of the areas of medicine previously discussed. In addition, phase 2 concludes after the candidate has shown a willingness and capability of leading a team through a call—by exhibiting the leadership qualities that were previously discussed.

Phase 2 also concludes when the candidate has shown consistent and reliable decision-making and patient advocacy. Phase 2 for most candidates with no experience or who are new to the role of paramedic should last approximately 400 hours. Some candidates will require much more time than this and some will require less. The candidate can now move on to phase 3.

6

Phase 3: Execution

Phase 3 of the field instruction process should be relatively short. Phase 3 should not consist of more than approximately 100 hours. It is a short phase in which the candidate can now reinforce all of the concepts that you have taught them.

During this phase they reinforce their understanding of medical principles and how to apply them in the field. They reinforce all of the leadership principles that were talked about in phase 2 and how to apply those in the field. During this phase they need to concentrate on providing consistent and reliable patient care and patient advocacy. In short, the candidate must consistently and reliably practice executing treatment plans.

By now the candidate should be operating almost completely independent of any input from the instructor. It is beneficial for the candidate to have around 100 hours of independent paramedic work with little oversight. What this does is reinforce to the paramedic candidate that they are capable of making sound decisions and good treatment plans and then executing them with the team.

During this phase you, as the instructor, fine-tune everything that you've already taught them. The vast majority of mentorship and instruction should be behind you. During this phase you begin to develop a new relationship with your student. The relationship that you develop is one of the four criteria for their final evaluation.

Final Evaluation

You are now at the end of the internship or field instruction. You've developed your methodical approaches with your student. You've created multiple teaching plans, simple and complex, implemented them, and executed them properly. You've measured their growth and understand that within those teaching plans they have met the objective and the goals within those objectives and they are now becoming successful.

But how do you measure whether or not a student is ultimately successful within the training process? You have to evaluate four specific principles to determine whether they can function as a paramedic independently. These four principles are as follows:

1. The candidate has to demonstrate a consistent and correct **understanding** and interpretation of the guidelines and protocols they work within, along with a consistent demonstration and understanding of medical principles. They must also demonstrate a consistent ability to perform the skills needed to provide care to patients (examples would be intubation and starting IVs).

2. During phase 3 the **relationship** should start to change from instructor/candidate to a peer-to-peer relationship. What this means is that your student's demonstration of decision-making should eventually get to a point where they are discussing their treatment plans with you on a peer-to-peer basis. This also goes hand-in-hand with their implementation of the methodical approach. This newfound relationship is demonstrating to you that the student is comfortable making decisions independent from your input and is confident in those decisions. This relationship is only developed after hundreds of hours of running calls and mentorship.
3. They have to demonstrate to you their **flexibility** in treatment plans. You want to be able to evaluate whether they can independently, without your prompting, change treatment plans in the middle of a call. They need to recognize the need for a change in treatment, develop a new plan, and implement the new plan during the call. This flexibility demonstrates the student's ability to reassess the patient, reevaluate treatment plans, and recognize when a new treatment plan has to be implemented in order to properly treat a patient that is changing.
4. Finally and arguably most important, the student must demonstrate their willingness to be **accountable** for the decisions they make. Accountability is key when they're functioning independently from you. You have to have confidence that they will hold themselves accountable for the decisions they make. This demonstrates the student's understanding of the side effects, consequences, risks, and rewards of the

interventions they perform. **Remember, the ability to make confident decisions is directly related to the individual's willingness to take responsibility for those decisions.**

If the student demonstrates these four principles, you, as their instructor, can be assured that they are probably very close to or ready to begin functioning as an independent paramedic.

Phase 3 is short. These principles should be focused on and reinforced:

1. Build confidence by consistently running calls almost completely absent from your input. This is very important for the candidate's development and shows them that they can function in this capacity.
2. Don't kneecap your candidate. This is incumbent on you to sit back and put your own ego in check and allow the candidate to run calls.
3. Fine-tune your candidate's decision-making. Go over specifics that they have questions about. Engage with them on a peer-to-peer status. If you have been successful, this new relationship is inevitable.
4. Ensure that they stay within local protocols or guidelines. This goes throughout the field instruction process. However, in this phase you should not interject yourself into a treatment plan unless it is violating guidelines. If you have been successful in your training of the student, this intervention should happen rarely, because you have impressed upon them the need to follow the medical director's intent, which is the guidelines and protocols.

We have concluded phase 3, which is short and sweet but highly important. If your candidate can pass this final evaluation, they are ready to work in the field independently.

Final Evaluation Form

1. Does the candidate demonstrate consistent and correct understanding of the medical principles as set forth in phase 2 of this workbook? Does the candidate demonstrate an ability to perform the skills needed (such as intubation and IVs)? If not, describe specifically what they do not understand (example: cardiology and 12 lead interpretation).
2. Does the candidate demonstrate an ability to change treatment plans on critically ill patients when they recognize something new or different in the patient? Are they flexible or are they rigid in treatment plans?

Give examples (such as incorporating a medical component into a trauma patient).

3. Are you able to discuss treatment plans with candidate on a peer-to-peer level? Or do you continue to need to intervene for safety and guideline purposes to make sure the candidate provides the standard of care to patients (example: During patient care are you discussing the treatment plan and options or are you needing to continually prompt for critical interventions?)?
4. Does the candidate demonstrate a willingness to be accountable for their decisions? Do they make excuses? Do they blame others for poor patient care or outcomes? Accountability of action is a direct reflection of an understanding of the potential consequences and/or benefit of the interventions performed and treatment plans implemented. Remember that this is an integrated approach, and candidates who demonstrate accountability and ownership of decisions also demonstrate a degree of understanding for medical principles because they recognize the need for implementing certain treatment plans and interventions. If candidate is not proficient, give specific examples.

About the Authors

Christian and Samuel Adams are identical twin brothers. They have over twenty years of combined experience responding to 911 calls. They both love working as firefighter/paramedics for the Colorado Springs Fire Department (CSFD), and they fervently believe in providing the highest quality patient care to the citizens of Colorado Springs.

Christian Adams is a Nationally Registered and Colorado State Certified Paramedic. He is also certified in RSI (rapid sequence intubation). In 2012 he was honored as the Pridemark/ Rural Metro Paramedic of the Year for the Denver metro area. He is trained and has worked with the CSFD TEMS (Tactical EMS) team and currently functions as a paramedic with the city's High Angle Rope Rescue team. He also functions as a paramedic preceptor for the CSFD.

Christian has an associate of arts degree from the New Mexico Military Institute and a bachelor's degree in criminal justice from the University of Northern Colorado.

When not responding to alarms, his favorite pastime is enjoying the Colorado outdoors with his wife and two boys.

†

Samuel Adams is a Nationally Registered and Colorado State Certified Paramedic. He is certified through the CSFD for RSI (rapid sequence intubation). He started his EMS career working as an EMT basic in the Denver metro area. After going through paramedic school, he worked in the Denver area as a paramedic responding to 911 calls. He is on the CSFD TEMS unit for the city (Tactical EMS). His current assignment is as part of the wildland firefighting deployment team for the Colorado Springs Fire Department.

In 2017 Samuel was named Paramedic of the Year for the Colorado Springs Fire Department. Sam also serves on a paramedic advisory committee for the CSFD, which advises the EMS system in Colorado Springs. Sam also works as a paramedic preceptor for the CSFD. He has an associate of arts degree from the New Mexico Military Institute and a bachelor's degree in criminal justice from the University of Northern Colorado.

His offwork time is spent with his wife camping in the summers and being around his two brothers.

Christian and Samuel Adams are the authors of *Life and Death Matters: Professionalism and Decision-Making for the First Responder* (2019), available on Amazon and at www.Field-Medics.com.

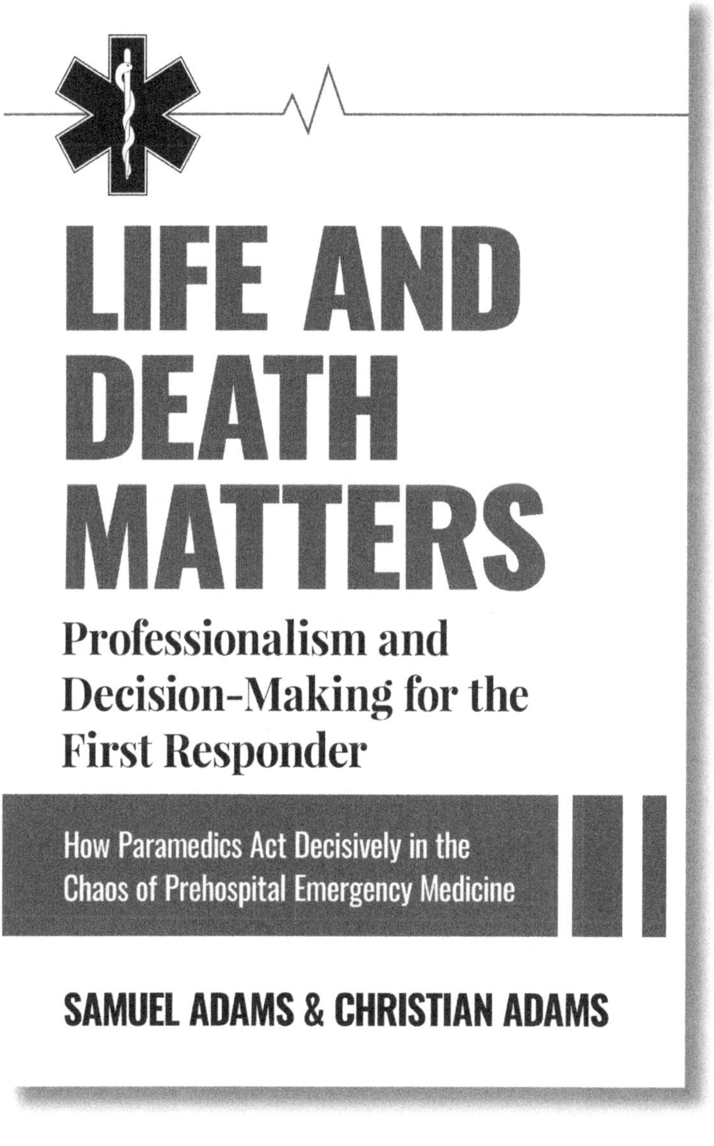
LIFE AND
DEATH
MATTERS
Professionalism and
Decision-Making for the
First Responder
How Paramedics Act Decisively in the
Chaos of Prehospital Emergency Medicine
SAMUEL ADAMS & CHRISTIAN ADAMS

Made in the USA
Monee, IL
04 November 2026

67385944R10066